Standing in the Doorway

*Stories of the dying
as witnessed by a hospice nurse.*

———————

by

Nona Harbert

Standing in the Doorway
Published by Total Fusion Press
6475 Cherry Run Rd. Strasburg, OH 44680
www.totalfusionpress.com

ISBN-10: 0990310000
ISBN-13: 978-0-9903100-0-6

Cover Design by www.fiverr.com
Edited by Andrea Long
Layout Design by Tina Levene

Library of Congress Control Number: 2014937995

Published in Association with Total Fusion Ministries, Strasburg, OH.
www.totalfusionministries.org

Scripture taken from the NEW AMERICAN STANDARD BIBLE®, Copyright © 1960,1962,1963,1968,1971,1972,1973,1975,1977,1995 by The Lockman Foundation. Used by permission.

Dedication

This book is dedicated to my mother Patricia, my father John, and my brother Perry. You opened my eyes to the sober joy of a soul passing through the doorway.

Preface

The names of my patients have been changed to protect their identities. I have deliberately kept their ages and hospice diagnoses vague for the same reason.

The photograph on page 72 is used by permission of the owner.

Table of Contents

Introduction

Caring for my dying father, and then my dying mother, taught me that death has certain patterns built into it—and that death is not what I thought it was. Just as a woman laboring to birth a soul into this world goes through predictable stages, so too does a body laboring to birth a soul into the next. While the stages of birth or death have predictable patterns, there is never a predictable story. You may linger in one stage of labor, almost slip past another, plateau for an indeterminate amount of time, and finally deliver a soul.

As a hospice nurse, I have witnessed every combination of soul birth stages I can imagine. Most of the caregivers I talk to understand intuitively that they are watching the dying process as they see their loved one eat less and less, sleep more and more, and distance themselves from normally-enjoyed activities. There are other behaviors that exhibit themselves closer to the end of life, and these are not as well understood. Reaching into the air while eyes are glazed over, asking for shoes, saying *it's time to go*, talking to deceased relatives, and asking if bags are packed are all examples of the end-of-life phenomenon. A hospice chaplain once explained it as the behavior of a soul standing in the doorway between earth and eternity: a person in a doorway can look behind them to the room they currently occupy, but also ahead to the place they are going. While families are grateful to be equipped to manage physical symptoms like pain and constipation, they report being most personally comforted by the explanation that de-mystifies these end-of-life behaviors.

I explained this "doorway perspective" to the family of an older gentleman. They listened politely but at least one family member had an openly skeptical look on her face. When I next visited, I was met by an excited, animated group with a story to tell: Dad had been minimally responsive all day, but suddenly threw his arms up and yelled, "Yee-haw! I'm going for a ride, here comes the train! Oh-no, I have to have a bowel movement; do you think they have toilet paper on the train?" A quick-witted son told his dad there was toilet paper on the train and that he should get on. His dad lay back in the bed with disappointment and said, "Oh no, I already went. I'll have to wait for another train." What a beautiful example of being present to both worlds! Two days later he asked if God had forgotten to send another train. A son who had been struggling to let go of him said with great sincerity it was time leave, and minutes later he died.

This book is written for all caregivers of those who are dying. I hope it helps and comforts you. We are holistic beings: physical, emotional, spiritual. My world view, and that of many of my patients, is a Christian world view. It may not be yours. I would encourage you to read these stories and strain them through your paradigm before you process them. My hope and intent is that you would be better equipped to be fully present to the dying as they are "Standing in the Doorway."

My Mom

My mom was loving, hardworking, and German tough. No whining, no crying for her when things got tough. When things were hard, you just tried harder. The factory she worked at produced fireplaces, and she was told to lift heavy boxes up above her head. Today no one would imagine that to be safe, but in the 1960s, OSHA was not present to protect her. When I was about twelve years old, she injured her back at work, causing extreme weakness in her legs and pain with movement.

I remember Mom going to great lengths to take care of herself during that injury: She would disappear into the bathroom to give herself an enema to have a bowel movement; piling clothes into a small laundry basket, she would sit on a step to the basement, slide down the steps to the laundry room, and come up again using her arms to pull her torso up. I don't remember her ever whining in front of us. The company doctor said that her x-rays were fine, and that there was not a problem. Her own doctor said she would probably never be better. She said she'd walk again.

Having eight kids was probably good therapy. Meals had to be made, babies rocked, and afore-mentioned clothes washed. As the years went by, her gait assumed more strength. Several springs later, a war whoop was heard from the driveway. There was Mom, riding a bike in a not-so-straight line down the driveway. I was happy for her, as happy as if she'd won an official race. Only an insider would know what price she'd paid to make that trip.

Years later, Mom faced a much harder battle. Cancer visited her, as it does so many people, and rudely refused to leave. She threw chemo at it, blasted it with radiation, and tried starving it. Meanwhile, cancer, this most unwelcome house guest, ignored her demands to leave.

Mom was living with me by this time. It was early spring, the time to get ready for Easter. Finding Easter baskets at our childhood house usually took seven hours or more. They were always full of chocolate and shredded colored grass and hidden well under a pile of clothes in the dryer, or inside a large plastic container on the top shelf in the kitchen cupboards. One of us was always begging candy from the others the last couple of hours, because everyone else had found their basket already. When we were close to crying, Mom would play "hot or cold" as we crawled through nooks and crannies in the house until we found our baskets. It seems there were always kids around who didn't have as much as we did, and yet we were probably poor by most people's standards. When it came to kids though, Mom had her priorities straight, and she always made sure that all the children in her world were cared for. We often made room at the table for someone who needed to belong somewhere for awhile.

That last year, Mom desperately wanted to help with Easter dinner. We settled on a nice meal planned for evening, when I got off work. I was a nurse on a busy step-down unit, and hoped to be home before 8:00 p.m., but plans changed. My husband called around 6:00 p.m., frantically explaining that Mom was having a seizure. I left work immediately, and arrived home twenty minutes later to find her shaking violently. She was able to make eye contact, skin gray and clammy, and her eyes begged me to help her. I didn't know how. I called Mom's hospice nurse, who arrived sometime later with a bottle of morphine and the intention of keeping us company as we waited for Mom to pass. She was nonresponsive by that time, no longer shaking and having periods of apnea. After an hour, little changed, I asked the nurse to leave. Mom had a strong heart and it almost seemed like her color and respirations were better. Fran, the nurse, left reluctantly. I settled down in a recliner to wait.

At 3:00 a.m. I heard my mother's voice saying, "Nona, I have to go to the bathroom."

"You do?" I replied, confused. "Do you remember anything about tonight?"

"No," she replied, "nothing."

I assisted her to the bathroom, happy to have her back, and dreading the time she would leave for good.

During the next few weeks, I watched her cut her ties with this earth, almost as if she was a hot air balloon with many ropes to be cut. She was still anchored here, but noticeably less and less with each passing day. Several times I found her lying in bed, reaching into the air and whispering something. When I would speak to her, she would turn her head slowly and look through me. She was taking on the eyes of eternity.

My brothers and sisters arrived for one last visit at the end of April. Mom's favorite part of the visit was watching the grandkids play and listening to us talk about our childhood. She did not join in, but I knew she was listening, even when her eyes were closed. We had an early birthday party for me, and I asked her if she would be here for my real birthday, May 4th. She looked me in the eye and said firmly, "I'll be there."

May 4th came and Mom was still here, struggling to stay awake for me. On May 5th, I knew she had set her sails for home. Only a few tiny ropes held her here. She would wake up briefly and respond appropriately, but I could see she was busy packing all the memories in boxes to take with her while her body continued its long, slow, shutdown. On May 7th, flowers arrived for her from my brother. He lives in the Seattle area, and had been here the end of April with my other siblings. I put the phone up by her ear so he could say goodbye, then called my other siblings to tell them that Mom's end was upon us.

I sat next to the bed until 3:00 a.m. when it seemed like an invisible, but peaceful force almost picked me up and walked me around the corner and placed me in the recliner. I thought to myself how strange it was that I was not panicked about leaving her. My eyes closed and opened three hours later. I ran to her room, and she was still with me, but the last few ropes that held her here had been cut. She could not do it with me sitting next to her. She had waited on the last rope so I could be with her. I had asked her weeks before if she would let me be with her when she passed and she said she would. I called hospice and requested Chaplain Paul to come. My husband, daughters, and son had all woken up by this time. They came in and said goodbye to Grammie. None of the kids wanted to be in the house when she passed, so they left for school, seeking refuge from the pain. Dennis, my husband, left to get a suction to try to get the mucous at the back of her throat. Chaplain Paul arrived minutes later, leaning down to Mom he said, "Pat, I'm here with Nona, you can go."

We waited thirty to forty seconds, and there was no breath. After another thirty seconds, we surmised that she had gone. What a Mom-like thing to do, waiting for back up before she left. Beautiful worship music filled the room. I turned the volume up as the words of "Agnus Dei" filled the room... *Alleluia – For the Lord God Almighty reigns! Worthy is the Lamb- Holy are you-Lord God Almighty!*

"The next day he saw Jesus coming to him and said, 'Behold, the Lamb of God who takes away the sin of the world!'" John 1:29

One week later we were in Wisconsin, where Taylor funeral home had hosted many a funeral for my family. Here we all were, one year after Dad died, doing it again. Many people went up to give honor to a life well-lived. Stories of children blessed by her presence filled the room. As the stories wound to an end, I had the director turn on the music. "Agnus Dei" swelled and floated and seemed to take on life, filling the room with praise. Tears flowed freely, but not all were of grief. The distinct smell of lily of the valley was discerned by many people to be wafting through the room. A feeling of deep, aching joy, followed by wonder, was reported from my sisters. What a fitting end for her. Dad had gotten a 21-gun salute when he left. Somehow I think he had a hand in making sure Mom was also properly honored.

"After these things I heard something like a loud voice of a great multitude in heaven, saying, 'Hallelujah! Salvation and glory and power belong to our God...'" Revelation 19:1

Having my dying mother in my home under hospice care, convicted me that God was calling me to a ministry with the dying, their families, and their care givers.

Getting on the Ship

My dear friend Nancy has another dear friend named Diane whom I see once a year at Nancy's birthday dinner. These two women are mighty in spirit, and I have heard God refer to them as his generals. When they speak, I listen, and when they pray, I follow their lead. These women are smart, filled with light and integrity, and are totally sold-out to God the Father, Jesus the Savior, and the Holy Spirit the Teacher.

At one of Nancy's yearly parties, I found myself asking Diane, "What was the most interesting thing you've seen this last year?" Her face became still as she reviewed her year, then she told me her amazing story. Diane works at a nursing home, often on the night shift. One of her elderly male residents was in poor health, and he asked to have his wife brought to him, as he was going to die today. Urgent phone calls resulted in his wheelchair-ridden wife being brought to his bedside. She leaned over him, grasping his hand, trying to find a way to say the painful, tender things we say at a deathbed. He mumbled something which made her ask, "Where are you?"

He told her he was standing on a shore, and he could see the ship coming. He paused and said, "That one's full—I'll wait for the next one."

She talked for several more minutes a
lay with his eyes closed. When she paused, he told
her another ship had come and she needed to let
go of his hand so he could leave. She did as he had
asked, and he promptly quit breathing.

I was much affected and moved by this
story, and asked Diane if she had ever seen one of
the "blue books" that our hospice gives to families.
(*Gone from My Sight: The Dying Experience* by
Barbara Karnes, RN.) The last page has a beautiful
poem by Henry Van Dyke which references a ship
being lost on our horizon, only to be hailed by a
welcoming crowd beyond our sight. She had not
read this book, but was intrigued by the similarity
of this man's story to the poem. I have heard many
other people announce they were going to leave,
but this was the only one who announced he was
sailing home.

*"I am standing upon the seashore. A ship at
my side spreads her white sails to the morning
breeze and starts for the blue ocean. She is an
object of beauty and strength. I stand and watch
her until at length she hangs like a speck of white
cloud just where the sea and sky come to mingle
with each other.*

*Then someone at my side says: 'There, she is
gone!'*

'Gone where?'

Gone from my sight. That is all. She is just as large in mast and hull and spar as she was when she left my side and she is just as able to bear the load of living freight to her destined port.

Her diminished size is in me, not in her. And just at the moment when someone at my side says: 'There, she is gone!' There are other eyes watching her coming, and other voices ready to take up the glad shout: 'Here she comes!'

And that is dying."

-Henry Van Dyke

Is the Kitchen Red Up?

I can't tell you much about Louise from firsthand experience. By the time I met her, she spoke very little and hardly ever a word to me. She saved her precious words for the people in her life who counted. It took very little tweaking to adjust her meds so she would be comfortable. The greater task was to help her husband and four daughters learn how to provide care to her now that she was bedbound, and how to have the resolve to finally let her go.

Several visits were spent dealing with the physical issues: Should we force her to eat? Why is her urine so dark? How often should her bowels move? Louise's family suffered anguish watching her "starve" herself. They often offered bites of her old favorites, only to have her say, "Maybe later…" I explained that Louise was not starving; she was getting ready to shut her body down.

Four daughters and a sad husband listened in silence, grief registering in downcast eyes and slumped shoulders as each one processed what I had just said. After a moment of quiet reflection, one of the daughters asked if her sister had heard Mom ask about the kitchen earlier.

"Oh, yeah," a sibling answered with a wave of her hand, "I don't know why she cares about the kitchen, but I told her we were cleaning."

"So what was she asking?" I said.

The sisters looked tolerantly at each other and smiled. Mom had asked if the kitchen was "red up." I wondered aloud why she cared about the kitchen—was that her private domain, or was she fussier about her kitchen then the rest of the house? Her daughters laughed, and then reported that Mom would never leave the house until the kitchen was "red up," as she hated coming home to a dirty kitchen. As the words left their mouth, I saw a look of understanding cross their faces, one after the other, like dominos falling. She was telling them something, and they finally heard it. When Louise went home two days later, her family was able to say goodbye.

Sarah

Sarah's daughter was meeting me at the nursing home to sign hospice admission papers. She had flown from Idaho to Ohio to get her mom settled in a safe environment. She reviewed the hospice program, signed necessary papers, and ensured that new orders were in place. Then Sarah's daughter asked me about what she really wanted to know, "How long?" I let her know that Sarah had a short time, to be measured only in weeks, probably not a month. Her daughter needed to know so she could take care of business at home, but also so she could begin to face the impending loss and process her grief.

Sarah's daughter wondered how I had come to my conclusion. I reviewed the signs and symptoms of a body shutting itself down: People quit eating meat several months before they die, as it is too hard to digest. They eat mashed potatoes, soup, cottage cheese, or pudding. Then they eat applesauce and sherbet, a few bites of something soft. Soon they just want sips of fluids, then refuse intake altogether. Sarah's daughter was initially horrified—we were letting her mother starve and dehydrate! *No, the shutdown of body is a slow and precise process*, I explained. We do not have to say to the dying, *it's time to quit eating meat*. They just know to do it. No one has to tell them what to eat—some internal gauge measures what can be digested and an invisible message is sent to the appetite center of the brain letting the body know what the digestive organs can handle. As months and weeks pass, the foods ingested become less and less complex, easing the strain off of a body trying to shut down.

The same thing with fluids, I continued to explain. As a weakened heart and kidneys struggle to handle the usual fluid load, intake magically decreases. In fact, the day before most people die, they are found in bed soaked with urine, much to their caregiver's surprise. The reason this happens is that our bodies inexplicably dump all the water they can, taking a load off the heart, so that fluid cannot overload the dying body and seep into the lungs. If you think about it, a cleaned out gut and a dry body present the most comfortable environment for the final shutdown. I have personally monitored dying bodies with tube feedings and IVs running; I have listened to gurgling respirations and cleaned up tube feedings squirting out from a peg tube. At the time, I didn't know better—I didn't feel like I could say to the families, or even the attending doctor, that the current treatment plan was causing distress. I was young, and had not seen many people die in a home environment where they could direct the intake of food and fluids.

"Deep calls to deep at the sound of Your waterfalls; All Your breakers and Your waves have rolled over me." Psalm 42:7

Another interesting thing happens as people are close to the end of this life. The Bible says that deep calls out to deep. Somehow, our soul knows we are getting ready to move before our conscious mind figures it out. This is often manifested as *travel language* in the dying. (For more on the concept of *travel language*, please read *Final Gifts* by Maggie Callanan and Patricia Kelley.) My mother would wake from a nap and ask if her bags were packed. She did not want to miss her train. I had a pilot ask if he had enough fuel to make it over, and an Amish man inquire if the buggy was ready. Many people lean forward, reaching into the air for unseen loved ones, murmuring, "I've got to go," or "I want to go home." As family reassures the dying member that they are home, they are missing the point. *Home* is not here.

The Temporal and the Eternal:
"(1) For we know that if the earthly tent which is our house is torn down, we have a building from God, a house not made with hands, eternal in the heavens. (2) For indeed in this house we groan, longing to be clothed with our dwelling from heaven, (3) inasmuch as we, having put it on, will not be found naked. (4) For indeed while we are

in this tent, we groan, being burdened, because
we do not want to be unclothed but to be clothed,
so that what is mortal will be swallowed up by
life." 2 Corinthians 5:1-4

The face of Sarah's daughter reflected a
strange, but familiar, mixture of wonder, pain, fear,
and hope. I turned to the pictures on the dresser
and asked about one with Sarah and a handsome
man. "That's my dad," her daughter replied. "Mom
and Dad met on a blind date. They had a picnic.
Daddy died just a few months ago." Condolences
were offered and I let Sarah's daughter know what
day I would be back.

My second visit found Sarah looking much
paler, sleeping twenty-two out of twenty-four
hours, and not even drinking much. The painful
transition from using a commode to a diaper had
occurred. Sarah's daughter was found in the
resident dining room. She was trying to read a
book, but looked sad and was easily distracted. She
could interpret her mom's physical changes and
knew her time was short. "I may try to fly home for
the weekend and clean up some things at work so I
can stay for Mom's end, and the funeral, without
causing problems at work," she reported. I
reminded her that Sarah's condition was slipping
pretty quickly. Her daughter said that she'd think
about it. I told her I'd be back in two days, and to
call if she needed us before then. When I returned

two days later, Sarah's daughter was there and met me in the hall. I verbalized a little surprise, thinking she might have gone home. The daughter told me she was sitting with her mom the day before, fully planning to go home for a day or two, when she heard her mom talking. Sarah could be heard saying, "I'm ready for my picnic." Her daughter knew who was meeting her for the picnic and decided to stay. Sarah went home during my visit that day—much quicker than any of us really thought. Her daughter, full of grief and wonder, got a close-up glimpse of a soul making plans to go home. She was grateful, and so was I.

Robert

I arrived at the older, beautifully restored home to be taken to a frail, thin man lying propped-up in bed fighting to breathe. His family was attentive, present, coping adequately, and willing to do whatever they needed to do to help him get comfortable. This family was sad and grieving, but not really frightened. They were not unfamiliar with death, but needed advice to keep him comfortable.

Hospice has very good tools for managing shortness of breath, such as oxygen, nebulizer treatments, and morphine. The greatest hindrance to achieving a patient's comfort is often the family's fear that using morphine will kill their loved one. The other treatments are usually well accepted, but the introduction of the small bottle of morphine drops is often met by fearful and anxious posturing, a slight backing up and shake of the head. "We're not ready for that yet..."

"We use small amounts... it is short acting... it is the drug of choice for shortness of breath..." I try to explain to the cautious family. But these explanations are often met with fear and skepticism.

Robert's severe dyspnea, or labored breathing, made his chest rise and fall in shallow, jerky movements about 30 times a minute. He had a C-Pap machine but did not like to use it. He kept his oxygen on through a nasal cannula without problem. He had breathing treatments, but did not use them consistently, and was not using anything for anxiety. I reviewed basic comfort measures with the family. As our conversation wandered, they began asking what it would look like when he died. They knew a little about how a body shuts down, but not much about what he would go through emotionally or spiritually.

I told them the parable I often tell people. If Robert was moving from this house to another, he would clean out his closets, drawers, and cupboards. He would sort everything, throw some things away, give some, and take some. I explained that his spirit and soul are getting ready to move, and they are doing the same thing. He will spend a lot of time with eyes closed—when you speak to him, he may not answer right away. If he does answer you, he may say something off the wall, or totally unexpected. When you repeat what you said to him again, he may look at you with clear eyes and give an appropriate response to your question or comment. The reason this happens is because his soul and spirit may have been twenty years deep in a memory closet, and he could not crawl out of it fast enough to be present to you. When his eyes are closed, he is not resting the way you think. He is packing up to move. Bob's family acknowledged they had witnessed this already, but had interpreted it as confusion or low oxygen.

I also told them about how we teeter between this world and the next until it feels right to leave. While this is happening, we get to peek ahead: we see glimpses of heaven and loved ones who've gone ahead. Bob's family digested this, admitting it was a surprise. They resolved to understand what he was going through to the best of their abilities.

Two weeks, and a frantic call later, I found myself gazing upon Bob's dying body. His condition had declined rapidly that day. Eyes half open, glazed over, skin pale and cool, I confirmed declining vital signs, and then gathered the family in the kitchen to help them process his passing to the next world.

His family had been talking openly and bravely with each other, and with Bob. His condition had been declining for weeks, and his imminent passing was expected. They reported being surprised he had been here as long as he was, considering the poor state of his health. They felt he had lingered due to fear of the unknown. Prayers had been offered for his peace and safety in eternity. Two of the family members present reported he had been reaching into the air the day before, and had called out to a favorite uncle. He told his family that the uncle was there with a dog he knew from childhood. Bob's family seemed to find comfort in this, and felt it made his transition easier to work through. He appeared quiet and peaceful when he left, and his family, though grieving, was comforted.

"Blessed are those who mourn, for they shall be comforted." Matthew 5:4

Ben

Sitting in a meticulously kept home, Ben and Eileen met me with both graciousness and skepticism. Ben's heart had been poor for years, why did he need hospice now? I talked with them about the convenience of having oxygen and morphine in the home to manage the ever-increasing frequency of angina attacks. He thought a minute, agreed he was sick of the emergency room, and answered my questions with patience and good-will.

Ben was a woodworker, and his porch was filled with bird houses he had made for the elementary school class his daughter taught. On one of my visits, I noticed the porch was empty and a bevy of homemade thank you cards was sitting next to his recliner. He grinned when I asked him about it. Ben loved to give.

He loved to visit his buddies for lunch, but as the weeks slipped by, these outings with friends became more cautious and required more planning, such as nitroglycerin pills, morphine drops, and portable oxygen. The heart-squeezing pain visited more and more often, and with greater strength. I could see his wife, Eileen, biting her tongue and holding her breath every time he talked about going to see the boys. His trips became shorter and less frequent. Brushing his teeth was enough to require medications, oxygen, and a two-hour period of recovery in the recliner. Several times I asked Ben if he had thought about where he was going, and what it might be like. He always nodded but never offered any thoughts on the matter. Most people verbalize fears or personal observations of what they have glimpsed, so I was led to assume these things were private to Ben— too private to share.

At this time, the holidays were upon us. Much to Eileen's surprise and frustration, Ben put a few spotlights up outside. They never got a tree up, but Eileen managed to whip up a few of their favorite cookies. Pain visited weekly, sometimes daily, and one day, came to stay. I visited Ben's house twice in one day. Unable to keep him comfortable with my tools and experience, I offered him an admission to our hospice house for symptom management. I told him he would have more expert management and better tools for pain, and it would give Eileen a chance to be his wife instead of his nurse. Eileen asked him to go, explaining she was afraid of the pain and felt inadequate to manage it. He said he'd think about it overnight.

I'm not sure if it was wrestling the pain all night or watching the fear and anguish in his wife's eyes, but Ben agreed to come into our hospice house by morning. It took several days to get him comfortable. He was obviously weak, short of breath, and afraid. I stopped to visit him on the days I worked; he always smiled and seemed to want to find something to laugh at, always looking to the light. On a Friday morning I asked if he felt peace about where he was going. His smile fading, he replied, "I don't know. I hope it is okay."

I left to go out into the community to see my other patients, and later received a phone call from the nurse at the hospice house. Ben's wife wanted to talk to me when I could make time.

I stopped by at the end of the day. Eileen was sitting on one side of Ben's bed; he lay back on the pillows, oxygen on, face pale, and voice weak. I decided to skip the small talk and ask Ben's wife if she was worried about where he was going. She looked at me with great sadness and said, "Yes." I asked him if he wanted to know how to go to heaven, and he told me he did. I looked at Eileen, not sure if she was comfortable with where the conversation was going, but she looked at me, very focused and alert, and nodded. I had the feeling this was something she had tried to share with him before, but perhaps he could not hear it from family.

"(1) In the beginning God created the heavens and the earth. (2)The earth was formless and void, and darkness was over the surface of the deep, and

the Spirit of God was moving over the surface of the waters." Genesis 1:1-2

I began the familiar story at the beginning. *The earth was created with goodness and life, and man was created in the image of God. All was peace, and health, and harmony. Meanwhile, in heaven, three archangels had been given much authority and power. Their names were Gabriel, Lucifer,* and then I paused. I couldn't remember the third angel's name, Eileen piped up with, "Michael!"

Yes, Michael! She looked at me and nodded as if to say, "Keep going!"

I continued the story: *Lucifer was trying to take over heaven, and took a third of the angels into revolt. They were thrown out of heaven and plotted a way to get even. They saw the beauty and vulnerability of God's creation, and began planning a way to bring death to it, for the wages of sin is death. It must have taken many years and much patience to find the right hook to snag Eve, for there were many generations of people on the earth by then. But one day was the right day, Satan, or Lucifer's, words fell on receptive ears, and sin opened the door for death to rush in. This was not a surprise to God, or his son, Jesus. They saw it coming and Jesus had a plan. They would woo back mankind and at the right time He would pay the wages of sin. Jesus would die, we could put all the sin on Him, and He would pay the cost.*

"The point of this, Ben, is you have a gift offered to you. Your sin is paid for; Jesus offers you the gift of life. The debt is erased—you just have to enter into agreement with Jesus that you are His and you accept the payment," I finished.

"(16) For God so loved the world, that He gave His only begotten Son, that whoever believes in Him shall not perish, but have eternal life. (17) For God did not send the Son into the world to judge the world, but that the world might be saved through Him." John 3:16-17

Ben looked at me, but remained silent. I thought he looked like was trying to process all this information. His wife hugged me and I said goodbye. I told him I would be back to see him after Christmas. The next afternoon, Christmas Eve, I got a call from a nurse in the hospice house. Ben wanted to talk to me privately, could I talk with him for a few minutes? Of course I could—they put me through to his room immediately. His wife answered and told me that Ben wanted to talk to me about something I said yesterday. She handed the phone to Ben and left the room.

"What did you want to ask me, Ben?" I asked.

There was a silent pause then a tiny small voice asked, "Would you help me know what to say so I can go to heaven?"

I asked him to repeat after me a simple, clear prayer thanking Jesus for the gift of life, asking Him to be the Lord of his life, and thanking God the Father for letting His Son do this wonderful, generous thing.

As Ben finished this prayer, I heard a soft sob, "Thank you, Nona."

"Thank you, Ben, and I'll see you on the other side."

Isabelle

A remarkably smooth face framed by perfectly brushed hair lay on the pillow, sending out to her family a message of peace and contentment. I never saw a moment's anxiety mar her placid countenance. Isabelle lay in a beautifully kept room in a beautifully kept home. Her Mennonite daughter, Carol, was efficient, confident, and calm. Very easy to be around, the daughter welcomed the support and knowledge that hospice brought into her home, but required very little physical assistance. She bathed her mom and tended to the minor breakdown in her skin without physical help. "Just show me what to do, and I'll do it," was Carol's mantra.

My visits to Isabelle were always like stepping into a calm oasis in an otherwise chaotic day. Sunlight poured through oak-framed windows, filtered by lace. An air ionizer provided the uplifting smell of fresh air, like the scent of the meadows surrounding a bubbling stream. The absence of electronic noise enveloped me and loosened my tense muscles.

Isabelle's unofficial diagnosis was "TMB," or too many birthdays. She did not have cancer, or heart failure, or renal failure, or emphysema. She just had a tired, elderly body. She spent most of her time lying perfectly still, almost appearing to be inert. I sometimes wondered why I was there. Her daughter, as caregiver, expressed appreciation for my support, and while I knew she needed the support, I always had a sense of being there to receive something, some unknown gift.

Weeks slid into months, and Isabelle's tiny body became smaller and frailer, taking up less and less room in the bed. Her face, however, never lost its aura of peace. Often a smile would simmer upon her countenance; but mostly her eyes were closed during my visits, as if I were not important to the task at hand. Most people need small amounts of morphine to ease the achiness of a body shutting down, but she required only a few doses in the entire time I knew her.

"In peace I will both lie down and sleep, For You alone, O Lord, make me to dwell in safety." Psalms 4:8

At the very end, Isabelle died the way she lived: quietly, without fanfare, without strife or anxiety, requiring little upkeep and with great dignity and grace. She was here, then left. Her essence seemingly floated from her shell on the breath of heaven. I was blessed to see a soul enveloped with peace. Perhaps I was not there for her as much as she was here for me.

"(16) Long life is in her right hand;
In her left hand are riches and honor.
(17) Her ways are pleasant ways
And all her paths are peace.
(18) She is a tree of life
to those who take hold of her,
And happy are all who hold her fast."
Proverbs 3:16-18

Veneta

Small and stately, with thick gray hair pulled back in a ponytail a teenager would envy, she met me at the door, her face lit up with a smile and dimples. Oxygen tubing sailed behind her and the hum of an oxygen concentrator leaked into the living room from the enclosed porch where she kept it. There was something regal about her as many people spontaneously testified. She even told me once that she had an uncle who was a member of the clergy in the King's court. Her children adored her and struggled to share her with each other in what was to be her last year with them.

Sent home to die, Veneta seemed unwilling to cooperate. A meticulous and well-schooled daughter helped Veneta to become more stable and comfortable, watched her diet, weight, and vital signs. A cardiac nurse could not have been more attentive or well-informed. Veneta grew a little stronger and her respirations become more normal as the weeks, and then months passed. She made it out to the mall a few times, and I thought perhaps I would be able to discharge her from the hospice program, but this was not to be. Symptoms that ranged from subtle to alarming appeared with increasing frequency, until every day became a struggle to find her way back to comfort. She was living alone in an apartment in an assisted living complex, placed there to provide a safety net for her in case she needed help when her children could not be with her. She particularly enjoyed the good company of shared meals and afternoon music performed for the residents. However, when she took enough medicine to be comfortable, she did not feel safe to walk around the building and join in the activities. Consequently, she often walked a very thin line between comfort and sedation and sometimes swayed to either side of that line in an attempt to keep her world together.

I would feel myself getting anxious as I parked my car in front of her building. I knew I would find her short of breath, still trying to live a life that included outings with her son, a glass of wine as she listened to someone singing songs from "her day," or a walk to the front patio with her new friends to watch the world coming and going. She would use the morphine once a day, twice if she were miserable, and refuse any more. I hated to see her labored breathing, but she knew what she wanted, and it was her life to live.

Several weeks into this struggle, Veneta's son called asking for an early visit. When I arrived, Veneta was sitting on the couch, her tiny peanut face pinched with anxiety. Skin pale and cool, fingers dusky, and speech slow, it made my chest hurt to see hers rise and fall with a rapid succession of quick, light breaths. Her son hovered at the kitchen table, looking like he was in over his head and surprised to find himself there, emotionally and physically overwhelmed. I made arrangements to admit her to our hospice care center and helped Veneta's son pack up her clothes and medications.

She was swiftly admitted to the hospice facility and word went out to all her children. The next two days found them arriving from several states, still working out some differences of opinion, but united in their love for their mother. Veneta held court from her bed with a minimum of words and an aura of love. She never said much, and when she did it was cloaked in grace and gentleness. She was one of many *grande dames* I have met in my life: centered, loving, and kind. She blessed me by just being. She blessed her children by letting them be who they had to be.

"(27) She looks well to the ways of her household,
And does not eat the bread of idleness.
(28) Her children rise up and bless her;
Her husband also, and he praises her, saying:
(29) 'Many daughters have done nobly,
But you excel them all.'
(30) Charm is deceitful and beauty is vain,
But a woman who fears the Lord,
she shall be praised.
(31) Give her the product of her hands,
And let her works praise her in the gates."
Proverbs 31:27-31

Mark

It was a gray, cold day as I approached the bi-level house with a confusing array of entries positioned at odd angels. An ambulance in the driveway was unloading a man in his forties on a cot, while his wife was busy trying to move furniture out of the way and direct them to a patio door at the back of the house. I followed the ambulance drivers in through the patio, assessed the room for available equipment and supplies, and found a table in a room at the top of a short flight of stairs to set up my hospice materials and computer. After the paramedics left, my prospective patient, Mark, fell into an uneasy sleep in his new hospital bed. His wife, Sherry, hovered nervously near the top of the stairs and paid minimal attention to my attempts to explain the hospice program. She was obviously afraid, processing grief, and hyper-alert as she watched her husband sleeping in the room below us.

As my conversation slid from information about hospice to questions about his condition, she began to focus more attention on what I was saying and slid onto the chair nearest the stairs. Sherry began to talk about how fast Mark had gotten sick, how surprised she was to find herself watching him lie in a hospital bed, and how unprepared she felt to be bereaved again. Her mother, she explained, had died two months ago.

She knew about hospice because her mother had received care from another hospice in our community. I felt better about the minimal attention she had given to my hospice routine, feeling she really was giving informed consent to the program.

She then began asking many questions about death itself, which is what she really wanted to know. *Why wasn't he hungry? Why weren't we putting an IV on him? Why was he so confused? Why was he reaching into the air? Why, why, why?*

I began the same explanation I had given hundreds of times before, and have given hundreds of times since: *His body was shutting down, food was no longer a necessity, but had become instead a burden: no one wanted to shut their body down with a gut full of undigested food. His kidneys and heart were slowing down also. He would gradually dry himself of fluids to take a load off his heart, which would help him at the end, because a heart burdened with a load of fluids often results in wet lungs.*

I did have one question still: "Are you sure Mark is really confused? What does he say that makes you feel this way?"

She replied, "He says a few odd things that don't make sense while he's sleeping."

I asked if he knew her and was aware of where he was. She felt he was oriented to person and place, but still making random, odd remarks. I began explaining the purpose of a life review, comparing it to getting ready to move, as I have many times in the past. I explained that when a soul is getting ready to move, it goes deep into the memory closets and pulls all the memories out and makes decisions about them. *Did I do well in this life, or could I have done better? Do I need to forgive, or be forgiven?* If you speak to someone who is decades back in a memory closet, you may get odd, seemingly non-relevant fragments or phrases as a response to your comment. As you ask again, "Can I get you anything?" Your loved one may look at you clearly and answer appropriately. The first random, confusing response was not truly confusion but just the clumsy attempt of someone trying to crawl backwards out of a decades-long closet full of memories. They could not do so fast enough to be fully present to you in the here and now.

Sherry seemed partially comforted by this, and looked at me fully, still with some anxiety lining her face, and asked why he was reaching into the air. His behavior had all the markings of hallucination or confusion. I explained that this was another end-of-life phenomenon. As we approach death, the veil between this world and the next is pulled back, and we get a glimpse of what lies ahead. I had observed many people close to the end, and shared with her some of the things they had told me. Most of them reported seeing loved ones who had gone before them. When I got to this part of my explanation, Sherry startled me by jumping out of her chair, running down the stairs, and saying loudly and bluntly to Mark, "Has my mother been here?"

His eyelids fluttered and he whispered, "Yes, she was here yesterday. Jesus was here too and He said He'd never leave me."

Sherry stood stock-still, staring at her husband. I could see the thoughts running through her head reflected in the minute changes of her expression, similar to the way a toddler's thoughts are all over his face as he learns a new task. Sherry turned to me after a few minutes and said, "It all makes sense now. I wished I would have known this when my mother died."

Mark lived only days after I met him, but he left me with a precious story I have shared with others, "He said He'd never leave me."

"Make sure that your character is free from the love of money, being content with what you have; for He Himself has said, 'I will never desert you, nor will I ever forsake you...'" Hebrews 13:5

"...and lo, I am with you always, even to the end of the age." Matthew 28:20b

Matt

I arrived at the front door of a lovely brick home in an upper-class neighborhood wondering about my new patient. A young man answered the door in response to my knock, wearing rolled-up shirt sleeves and jeans. He was breathing a little hard as I entered and sat in the offered chair in the kitchen. He offered me something to drink, and then sat down for the interview. This was my new patient.

He was painfully thin with bright eyes, quick wit, and an air of gracious kindness covering him like a mantle. He came from a financially privileged home, but he did not seem to take his privilege for granted. I had never met a man who enjoyed serving others as he did.

The summer went by fast, as it always does. I visited him several times a week as we worked on ways to manage his shortness of breath and talked about the life he had lived. He spoke lovingly of his wife and son many times with pride at their accomplishments. He never mentioned what their lives would be like without him, but made quiet plans to sell a second vehicle and ensure the bills would be paid after he was gone.

"For he will never be shaken;
The righteous will be remembered forever."
Psalms 112:6

One cool night that fall, his wife called me to come look at Matt. She feared he was dying and wanted my opinion. I found Matt lying on the couch, as small and frail as a teenager going through a growth spurt. Eyes closed, his breath became irregular, sometimes with long pauses between breaths. His skin was cool and pale, and his blood pressure was very hard to hear. He had all the earmarks of a body shutting down. Matt had evoked both genuine respect and affection in all who knew him, including me. I gently lifted him so his wife could slide a waterproof pad under him in case he was incontinent. This had been his greatest fear, that his wife would witness him incontinent. He had refused a hospital bed, with all its implications of a diseased body, and had slept on the couch for weeks, propped up on pillows.

After talking with his wife about disease process and comfort measures, I knelt beside him and told him goodbye. I let him know how honored I felt to know him, what an example of love and grace he was, and what an obvious impact he had on our community. I kissed his forehead and whispered, "I hope you're at the gate to meet me when it's my turn to come home." Matt's eyelids fluttered, and I knew he had heard me.

As I drove away it occurred to me that he might need a medication to dry his respiratory secretions. After contacting the doctor and receiving the order, I called Matt's home to speak to his wife. A man answered the phone, "Hi Nona, it's Matt. I heard every word you said but I couldn't speak. I'll be there to meet you when it's your turn."

I was silent for a full ten seconds as I struggled to process what I had just heard. A few inadequate sounds escaped my lips before I asked for his wife. She heard my instructions regarding the medication for secretions, and then excused herself from the phone to lift Matt onto the bedside commode. He voided one last time and later died continent and respected, before the wife he adored.

"Delight yourself in the Lord;
and He will give you the desires of your heart."
Psalms 37:4

Matt was granted his last request, and in typical generous Matt fashion, left me a gift that I often pass on to others. Any hospice employee will tell you with full confidence that a person leaving this earth hears everything to the end. But Matt woke up and proved it.

Henry

Sitting in his recliner by the front window, Henry watched the cars go by and kept an eye on the goings-on in his living room. His tidy, sweet wife had a bit of dementia, but kept their home going with support from a loving and conscientious daughter. Henry was dealing with cancer, and had intermittent bouts of confusion himself, but always spoke to me appropriately when I conversed with him.

His daughter was so good to her parents, sacrificial of her time, and never complained about the "burden" of their care. They, in turn, seemed to trust her. This was a healthy family. I heard many stories about Henry, his love for his own children, as well as his nieces and nephews. Yearly vacations with Henry were favorite memories amongst the now-grown children in his family. He was the favorite uncle, and a beloved father. He'd lived a full life, and now it was drawing to a close.

The last six weeks or so, Henry began reporting bad dreams. His daughter felt he was sometimes awake and hallucinating at night. She reported that several times he called out, "The flames! The flames!" I felt uneasy, not sure if he was hallucinating or perhaps seeing a bit into another world. Patients often report glimpses of either a good place or a place of flames. Since

Henry had no avowed religious belief system, I didn't feel free to question him too closely. His doctor was notified, Haldol was ordered, and yet the hallucinations continued.

I arrived one day to find Henry sitting in his favorite chair by the window. His daughter was sitting in the dining room at the table. I sat down by her, began the usual litany of questions regarding medications and bowel movements, when we heard Henry yelling in the next room, "I'm going to hell if I don't change my ways!"

His daughter's face registered a mixture of confusion and amusement. It was going to be one of those days. I continued to ask more questions about pain and diet. Again we heard him, words thrown across the room like a whip, "I'm going to hell if I don't change my ways!"

His daughter's face registered less amusement and more confusion. I asked her if she had talked to him about his fear.

"No, he's a good man, I never really took it seriously," she answered.

I asked if she minded if I talked to him since he seemed so upset. She shrugged her shoulders and said, "No, I don't mind, go ahead."

**"Do not fear those who kill the body but are unable to kill the soul; but rather fear Him who is able to destroy both soul and body in hell."
Matthew 10:28**

Henry's worried face relaxed minutely as I approached, as if he hoped I could help him or at least would just be close to him in his fear. I began with a straightforward question, "You're worried you're going to hell?"

"Yes," he replied with great firmness and a lowered voice.

I asked if he believed in God, Jesus, heaven, and hell. He replied that yes, he did believe in all of that. I asked if he understood how it all worked, and he replied that he did not understand, but wanted to. I looked up at his daughter in the next room. She was standing now, close to the door and listening. I waited and watched her face, she gave no clue as to what she was thinking, and I knew I needed to seek her consent before getting in any further.

With his daughter's permission, I then shared this story with Henry: *God made the earth and all that was in it without sin, and without death. Adam and Eve were created. God loved them and they loved God. They trusted and obeyed Him and had everything they needed to live a life in*

Paradise. The Lord often spent time with them in the day. Sometime before this, a great battle had occurred in heaven, one of the three archangels decided he wanted the power of being God and talked a bunch of the angels into joining him. They got thrown out of heaven.

"And the great dragon was thrown down, the serpent of old who is called the devil and Satan, who deceives the whole world; he was thrown down to the earth, and his angels were thrown down with him." Revelation 12:9

This archangel, Satan, hated God and wanted revenge. He couldn't hurt God, directly, so he plotted to hurt his children. Adam and Eve had everything, and all that freedom had to offer in Paradise. The only thing God withheld from them was the fruit of the tree of knowledge of good and evil. I'm not sure what was in the fruit, but it is reported that eating it allowed them to have knowledge of good and bad, where before they must have only had knowledge of good. Satan came to Eve and worked on her until she gave in and ate of the fruit, and encouraged Adam to do so also. The minute they disobeyed, sin entered into them and also into the earth. The contract to live in paradise was over, and a new contract was made. This new contract read: the wages of sin is death.

"For the wages of sin is death, but the free gift of God is eternal life in Christ Jesus our Lord." Romans 6:23

Satan thought he had won. He had hurt God by hurting his children and bringing death to them and to the earth. God the Father had so much love for us and our world, that when his son Jesus said that He'd pay for it, God let him. Jesus took the sin—all of it from all the ages—and died with it. The wages were paid. Satan probably shrieked with the glee of winning when he saw Jesus die, but what he did not know was that God took his mighty arm and raised Jesus from the dead.

"If we confess our sins, He is faithful and righteous to forgive us our sins and to cleanse us from all unrighteousness." 1 John 1:9

The new contract offered to us says: if you believe in the gift of life Jesus offered to you, and confess it with your tongue you may go to heaven. He paid the wages of sin with his life, and he offers you the way into heaven.

Henry looked shocked. I expected him to look at least skeptical or confused. This was, after all, an amazing story. Looking me straight in the eye he said, "That's a good deal."

Smiling, I replied, "It sure is, Henry. Do you want in on it?"

"Yes!" he replied. Together we prayed a simple prayer of acceptance and thankfulness for the gift of eternal life in Jesus.

Between that day and the end of his life on this earth, we did not hear anything else about flames. Henry never talked about that day or my story again. He was intermittently vague to slightly confused, but I never sensed fear from him after that. Struggle and angst were absent at the end. He was observed reaching into the air, as so many people do. I don't know who he was reaching for, but I wish I did.

Polly

Nursing homes are not counted among my favorite places—big surprise. We all wish we could be home with family at the end of our lives. Unfortunately, many families lack the resources, either physical or emotional, to care for the chronically ill at home. Such was the case with Polly. Passing middle age and just sliding into her senior years, she was a resident in a facility. The staff gave good hands-on care and several staff members made it a point to stop in her room and visit with her. She probably was one of a handful of residents with a really clear mind and was able to converse intelligently.

Polly had one daughter who lived locally. She worked full-time and was up to her eyebrows taking care of her children. Polly really had nowhere to go, but she never felt fully at ease in the nursing home. Even though she complained of anxiety, she would only take medication to help her deal with it intermittently. It was worse at night when she was more alone. If I visited her in the morning, I was apt to find her lying in bed with the door closed. She reported poor sleep due to not being able to turn her brain off, and fear of what was to come.

I arranged visits from ancillary staff. Hospice is lucky to have pastors, social workers, counselors, massage therapists, and music therapists to help a soul find peace as the end draws near. Polly declined most of these services, however, deciding to only try the massage therapy. Weeks went by, and Polly continued a slow decline. Her daughter visited often, and Polly brightened up briefly when she was with her, and then reverted to her baseline of fear and anxiety.

One cold, damp, misty morning, I walked into the facility feeling frustrated and helpless, knowing Polly was declining and unwilling to let go because of fear. Her room was dark in the morning light, and a look of anxiety and pain lined her face. Skin pale, her eyes were closed with dark bags under them. Her primary nurse reported that Polly had a restless night but was unwilling to be medicated. I asked her if she was afraid to die, not because I was unsure of her response, but because she needed to talk.

Averting her eyes, Polly replied with a *yes* to my question. She didn't offer anything else, and I wasn't sure what else was going to be communicated. I asked if I could pray for her and she both nodded and looked eager to have me do so. She took my offered hands and held them, holding on as if to a lifeline. I prayed, "Father, let this woman know deep in her heart and mind what she means to You. Let Your love for her be real, and let her know You will keep her and care for her. Please let this happen in a way that is real to her. Amen."

Polly cried a little, thanked me, and closed her eyes, dismissing me from her room.
Three days later I returned. Her eyes were still closed, but her face no longer looked anxious. All the worry lines were gone and she actually looked younger. I spoke her name and she responded, but did not open her eyes. Her voice was weaker; she was not eating and slept most of the time.

"Polly," I asked, "what happened? You don't look afraid anymore."

She whispered quietly but clearly, "I walked in heaven."

Now she had my attention. I greedily craved details. Of course I heard what I always hear, "It's beautiful."

Feeling a strange mixture of relief and disappointment; I finished my physical assessment and tried one more time. "Polly, what was heaven like?" But she did not answer. "Polly, are you still afraid?"

"No," she replied, respirations unchanged. Polly left this earth about a week later, taking the information I coveted with her.

Marie

Sitting six feet from me was a plump woman, 95-plus in years, suffering from dementia as well as vision and hearing loss. She was blessed to be living with a super-attentive daughter and son-in-law. Marie's daughter was telling me about an episode that had occurred between nurse visits. "Mom was only breathing five or six times a minute and was unresponsive. Her color was almost white and her skin was cool to the touch. It lasted about thirty minutes, and then she opened her eyes and said, 'I'm still here.' She seemed surprised, so I asked her where she had been. 'I've been walking in Heaven. Jesus was with me. He held my hand and was very kind. He said I had to stay here awhile.'"

Marie's daughter was looking at me and requesting a response with her eyes. I asked if this had happened before and was told that it *never* had. Marie seemed fine—not upset by it at all—so we decided to take it at face value and see what happened.

Months and months went by, and finally a year passed. Marie was not so plump, even harder of hearing than before, and needed to be lifted from the bed to a recliner for her morning routine of coffee and oatmeal. She did not make any more heavenly trips, but had taken on the habit of conversing with many of her deceased relatives. Every nurse visit I got a run-down on who had been there to see Marie. She always looked up, smiled, and told her daughter who was visiting. Her poor daughter was not enjoying the family reunion so much, and often seemed flustered as she gave me the latest updates on these mysterious visitors. She had read our little blue book which talked about being close to death. The book explains that many people teeter with a foot in this world and a foot in the next; rocking back and forth until the day it feels comfortable to leave. This seemed to comfort Marie's daughter, as she felt more like her mom was the visitor, rather than all the deceased relatives.

As we were partially into Marie's second year with hospice, I noticed Ron, Marie's son-in-law, looking weak, pale, and tired. His wife voiced worry and concern, wondering whether he needed to see a doctor. Several weeks later, I arrived at a house full of turmoil. Ron was in the bedroom, confused, incontinent, and unmanageable. Marie was in bed but not sleeping. Her daughter was trying to get Ron into the bathroom. He would have none of it. An ambulance had been arranged to pick up Ron and take him to the hospital for evaluation. Several problems were found, the most devastating being colon cancer.

I have never seen a caregiver so brave or so tired. Marie's hospital bed was in the living room. Ron's was in the dining room. Two months of shuffling between rooms, even with the extra help she had hired, left Marie's daughter numb and exhausted. Oddly enough, Marie's daughter seemed to draw comfort from the fact that Marie was still with her, asking in one breath why her mom was still with her, yet appearing anxious and calling her mom back every time she got to close to leaving. Several times Marie quit breathing and lost her pulse during a routine nurse visit, but her daughter always shook her arm and yelled, "Mom! Mom!" and Mom came back.

As the end drew near for Ron, his daughters were present and his wife abandoned her mom to give full attention to her husband. By now Marie was cachectic, frail, with tissue paper skin over tiny little bones. She would sometimes whisper: *Who is that poor woman lying down there in that bed?*

The lovely cool evening was well advanced when Ron went home. Gentle tears and laughing/sobbing goodbyes followed him from this world. As the family drew close to his body, I discreetly retired to another room to give them privacy. I leaned over to make sure Marie was breathing and I heard her speak clearly, "Ron's gone." I asked her how she knew, but she couldn't tell me.

The daily visits from long-lost family members continued for Marie, and the day after Ron passed, Marie looked up in surprise and said, "Ron, you're here!" Such bittersweet words had never been heard by her daughter. Ron was "here" but he was not *here*.

Ron's funeral came and went, but Marie stayed on in this world. She was not eating, barely drinking, barely living, but still fully here. Several more months passed. The television was on and a commercial came across the screen promoting something none of us cared about. The twice-weekly litany of questions about intake and bowel movements, numbers of wet diapers, and quality of sleep was in full session, when Marie finally spoke. Softly we asked her to repeat what she said. Marie responded, "On the TV there..." and began reading the screen to us. Her daughter asked her to repeat it, and in a very rare moment of lucidity, she did. She read all the print—even the smallest words. Marie could not even identify me eighteen months ago as her vision was so poor, but she could now read the TV at the other end of the room. I had experienced other patients whose hearing seemed to improve when they were close to the end, but I had never seen or heard of this extreme vision improvement.

"Lord, make me to know my end
And what is the extent of my days;
Let me know how transient I am." Psalms 39:4

Two years after she walked with Jesus, Marie went home for good. It was finally all right with everyone for her to leave. Numbness encompassed her daughter as tears washed her soul. There would be no more hospital beds in her home, no more diapers, or straws, or pills crushed up in applesauce. I was never exactly sure what was accomplished in heaven or on earth by her extended stay, but it must have mattered, or Marie could have left a lot sooner.

Eva

A fair-haired woman with a heavy body and a manipulative spirit filled the bed and the living room of the tiny house. Eva was bedbound, but still controlled the goings-on in her home. Her two sons had moved in to care for her the last few months, determined to keep her from a nursing home. Eva engaged me in pleasant-enough conversation when I visited, offering a thank-you when appropriate, and calling out, "Have a nice day!" when I left. Her sons did not have it quite so good. They always appeared haggard and weary when I arrived. During my visits, they would talk with me in the kitchen in a low voice, glancing toward the living room to see if she might be listening. She would sometimes call out to them, and if they did not answer right away, she would escalate volume, frequency, and tone until she got her needs met. When I would prompt her sons to respond, they paused, and then explained that this was an on-going, all-day, everyday behavior. They reported that no matter what they did for her, minutes later it would be forgotten, not good enough, or wrong. As several weeks passed, I could see that family reconciliation was going to be one of our major goals of care. At least several times, I found one of her sons outside crying, smoking a cigarette, trying to muster the courage to go back inside.

Both sons talked openly about their spiritual concerns for their mom. It really bothered them that she just didn't get it. Eva loved to have scripture read to her, and quoted it on occasion. It did not seem to have changed her heart much, however. Her sons reported she had spent most of her life immersed in wild parties, drugs, sex, and miscreant friends who had used her. When I asked her sons what they wanted from hospice, they replied that they wanted us help them manage her symptoms, teach her to be patient with them, and to help her to have a good death. More weeks went by, Eva's physical symptoms were managed, and massage therapy and clergy visits were in place. Eva seemed restless and irritable at times. On several occasions I heard her speak to her sons with foul language and anger. They looked like whipped puppies when this happened, yet it never seemed to affect their caregiving. When I would mention to Eva how lucky she was to have sons who were so devoted to her, Eva would turn her head away from me and look angry.

During one visit, Eva's son sat down in the kitchen and haltingly reviewed the events of the previous night. He had heard his mom arguing with Jesus. This went on for hours. Jesus had apparently left, and Eva began screaming at her sons to get the keys for the door: "He went through the door and it's locked, I can't open it! Get me the keys!"

I called our hospice chaplain and filled him in. He visited within a few days and Eva told him about the closed door. She asked our chaplain for the keys. He asked her directly what kind of key she thought might open the door. Eva, however, would not answer him. He talked with her about Jesus having the keys of life.

"Then I will set the key
of the house of David on his shoulder,
When he opens no one will shut,
When he shuts no one will open."
Isaiah 22:22

During my next visit, I was again talking with one of her sons. He reported feeling frustrated and fatigued by her constant nagging for the mysterious keys. She never let up, and he had run out of ways to try and divert her attention. As I was listening to him, a scripture came to mind:

"The Lord is nigh unto them that are of a broken heart; and saveth such as be of a contrite spirit."
Psalms 34:18 (King James Version)

When I had a chance, I spoke this scripture to Eva and asked her what it meant to her, but she did not reply. Later that afternoon I ran into the hospice massage therapist. She told me Eva was as hard on her sons as ever. Apparently, our massage therapist had asked Eva if she knew what it was to have a contrite heart. Astonished, I asked if she had really used the word contrite, and if that was a word normally used in her vocabulary. The therapist answered that yes, she had said contrite, but no, it was not one of her normal words. I related my conversation from that morning; we both expressed feeling peace that God was working in her life.

Almost three full weeks passed before Eva left this earth. The family had tapes of scripture playing. Eva seemed to draw comfort from this. At the end, she slipped away peacefully, with no struggle, anxiety, or fear. Her sons had the satisfaction of knowing they showed up for her with love and integrity. They feel that the door was open to her at the end, and I agree.

**"Behold, I stand at the door and knock;
if anyone hears My voice and opens the door,
I will come in to him and will dine with him,
and he with Me." Revelation 3:20**

Martha

The nursing home called me, requesting a nurse visit for Martha. She was sitting bolt upright in a chair, refusing to go back to bed, and refusing to close her eyes. Her nurse at the facility felt she needed stronger anxiety medication. When I went in to visit her, I suspected she was afraid, and with good reason. She had the kind of fear in her eyes that a little tranquilizer was not going to fix. As I faced her family, very traditional in appearance and manner, I wondered how to talk with them about what I was seeing. We walked to a vacant lounge, sat down, and I inquired about their belief system. They belonged to a mainline, protestant church.

"Well," I asked, "what do you know about Satan?"

They looked uncomfortable, glanced warily at each other, and said, "Not much."

They did believe in him but did not know much about him. I explained what I knew from the Bible. *Satan is a prowling lion—he goes after the old, the sick, and the weak. Fear is his greatest weapon, and lying is his native tongue.*

"Be of sober spirit, be on the alert. Your adversary, the devil, prowls around like a roaring lion, seeking someone to devour." 1 Peter 5:8

"You are of your father the devil, and you want to do the desires of your father. He was a murderer from the beginning, and does not stand in the truth because there is no truth in him. Whenever he speaks a lie, he speaks from his own nature, for he is a liar and the father of lies." John 8:44

"For our struggle is not against flesh and blood, but against the rulers, against the powers, against the world forces of this darkness, against the spiritual forces of wickedness in the heavenly places." Ephesians 6:12

I continued on: *The reason it is important to know this is that when people are at the end of their lives, Satan will often come as a bully and torment them as they work out the last details of their life. Most people have forgiveness issues to take care of at the end, and Satan will torment them with fear and lies and cause them to lose their peace. It is important to help the dying by giving them a clean spiritual environment to work out their issues.*

Many glances passed between family members and I thought I'd perhaps gone too far. Finally, Martha's daughter spoke. She reported that she had spent the night in her mom's bedroom and had felt an evil presence. She refused to sleep there again. She then related that her brother had arrived from out of town and the same thing had happened to him.

The brother quickly denied it, saying, "No, no, no—that is not right. That's not what happened!"

His dad was present and spoke firmly, "Yes, this did happen, but what we can do?"

I reviewed briefly what scripture says about music in warfare. Before the Israelites went out to battle, they sent the choir out to sing praises. When King Saul was tormented by demons, he would call for David to sing praises and play his harp. The demons always left—they could not stand the sound of praise. The Psalms actually talk about praise shackling spiritual enemies in high places—it is no wonder why God told the choir to precede the army!

"(21) When he had consulted with the people, he appointed those who sang to the Lord and those who praised *Him* in holy attire, as they went out before the army and said, 'Give thanks to the Lord, for His lovingkindness is everlasting.'
(22) When they began singing and praising, the Lord set ambushes against the sons of Ammon, Moab and Mount Seir, who had come against Judah; so they were routed."
2 Chronicles 20:21-22

"So it came about whenever the evil spirit from God came to Saul, David would take the harp and play it with his hand; and Saul would be refreshed and be well, and the evil spirit would depart from him." 1 Samuel 16:23

"(5) Let the godly ones exult in glory; Let them sing for joy on their beds.
(6) Let the high praises of God be in their mouth, And a two-edged sword in their hand,
(7) To execute vengeance on the nations And punishment on the peoples,
(8) To bind their kings with chains And their nobles with fetters of iron,
(9) To execute on them the judgment written; This is an honor for all His godly ones. Praise the Lord!" Psalms 149:5-9

Martha's family joined me in prayer with her, asking for angels to protect, the blood of Christ to cover (demons hate that), and the Holy Spirit to fill her room. With a sigh, Martha's body went limp, her eyes closed, and she lay back in her chair. Her husband went home to get some worship music to play in her room. No medications were needed, just a clean room for her to finish her life work. She died within days, and she died in peace.

Maggie

It was a cold, rainy, on-call night. If you're a hospice nurse, you know the kind of the night I mean. It's the night you lay in bed and beg God to keep everyone comfortable and asleep until 8:00 a.m. I don't know why I pray that—He always does what he wants, anyway. On this particular night, the phone rang around 2:00 a.m.

Maggie was eighty-four and dying, currently sitting bolt upright in her bed with her back against the high headboard. Her caregivers were two adult nieces. Maggie had never been married nor had any children. She had lived alone until the last month when her nieces moved in. They sat in the kitchen looking scared. Maggie was in the bedroom screaming into the air, "I won't go with you... you can't make me... I refuse to die!"

A quick assessment was performed. She was within days of death, afraid, and not wanting anyone's help. I asked her if I could pray with her—NO was her firm answer. She told me I could hold her hand, though, and sit with her. This went on for 10-15 minutes, until I wrestled my hand away from her to go talk to the nieces. When asked how I could help them, they told me they were exhausted from sitting with her. They also feared she had not chosen well regarding eternity. Maggie had been angry with God, and had not shown interest in anything spiritual for as long as her family remembered. They requested I pray with them.

"For where two or three have gathered together in My name, I am there in their midst."
Matthew 18:20

As we reviewed what we knew about prayer, we realized Jesus was present when two or more gathered in His name. He was faithful, and would allow Maggie to stay long enough to make an informed decision. We prayed for her tormented soul, and I went outside to gather some supplies and paperwork for her respite admission into the hospital. While I was outside, I paused to pray in the spirit a few minutes. When I came back into the house, I heard Maggie yelling, "Come pray the Lord's Prayer with me!"

"(9) Pray, then, in this way:
'Our Father who is in heaven,
Hallowed be Your name.
(10) Your kingdom come.
Your will be done,
On earth as it is in heaven.
(11) Give us this day our daily bread.
(12) And forgive us our debts,
as we also have forgiven our debtors.
(13) And do not lead us into temptation,
but deliver us from evil.

[For Yours is the kingdom and the power and the glory forever. Amen.]'" Matthew 6:9-13

What a turn-around! Her nieces went in and prayed with her. They talked about God's immeasurable love for her. They shared His gift to her, all the debt that was paid for through the blood of his Son, and her need to accept that gift if she desired to live with Him. Maggie was surprisingly quiet, no longer belligerent or afraid. The last time I saw her she was leaving the house on a cot steered by the ambulance drivers.

I believe that what Maggie saw when I first arrived at her home literally scared her into heaven. I called her nieces after she passed and they reported that Maggie died peacefully, no more fear or screaming. They felt good about her passing, with no evidence of things to be feared.

God Sent Valentines

One of my coworkers was off work one gray damp day early in February. Two inches of soggy snow lay on the ground. One of her families called in to report that the patient, Bill, had a condition change and needed a nurse visit. My schedule was light, so I took the call.

Bill lived at the end of a cul-de-sac. His long driveway and cul-de-sac were pristine, white with snow. I parked on the road, unsure if anyone in the house needed to leave, not wanting to block the driveway. Bill's wife met me at the door, anxious, fearful, and fatigued. Bill was restless and unsteady, short of breath, and a little confused. His heart was failing, and he had only weeks to live by the looks of him. A telephone call later, I was on my way to the pharmacy to pick up morphine to use in addition to his oxygen.

Morphine in hand, I returned to the house, and decided to save my shoes and pull up into the driveway. Bill's wife met me at the door again, this time asking me excitedly if I had done that for her. Not knowing what "that" was, I stared at her and tried to figure out what she was talking about. She finally understood that I was clueless, and pulled me to her front picture window. Out on the road in the cul-de-sac were two beautiful hearts intertwined. They would only last as long as the snow, but Bill's wife had a perfect shot of them framed in her picture window. My tires had apparently made the hearts. Of course I had no idea how I'd done it or how to duplicate them. I did have a real sense, however, that they were meant as a gift to Bill's wife, a personal touch to comfort her and remind her of a bigger love.

A few weeks later, on February 14th, Bill went home. We're told that a bird cannot fall from heaven without His knowing; he obviously lives outside of time and knows the day and hour His children are arriving home. I even believe He arranges a special welcome for them. I was very touched by His acknowledgement of one woman's loss; valentines in snow for His special girl.

"Are not two sparrows sold for a cent? And yet not one of them will fall to the ground apart from your Father." Matthew 10:29

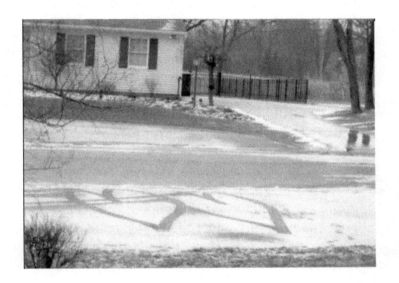

Born from Grief:
My Story

At age 15 I used to pray: *Please don't let our house burn down and don't let anyone in my family die.* That year was painful. My grandfather and a close uncle died in the spring; one of a stroke and the other of a heart attack. That summer a girl I knew from school was killed when a car hit her. My mother was pregnant with her eighth child, and on the fall day that she delivered her, a boy I knew from school died in a hunting accident. The same day, a neighbor, whose children we ran and played with, fell dead of a burst aneurysm.

My deceased uncle had two sons, and the deceased neighbor had one son in the same age group as my four younger brothers. These boys had built many a fort and rode many miles on their bikes together. Now three boys in this group were fatherless.

My own father was a construction worker. He was good at his craft, hard-working and reliable. People counted on him and were grateful for his skills. Many job sites asked for him to come back and do touch up work because they knew he would get it done right. Unfortunately, my father was also an alcoholic, and for the first time in my memory, construction was slow that year and he was laid off. In the first few weeks of no work, he drank quite a bit. After that, the habit waned. There probably wasn't the money for it. We would often go to his newly-widowed sister's house, and my brothers and her two young sons would spend hours together, getting into, or trying to avoid, trouble.

One February afternoon during a visit to my aunt's house, my father insisted that his sister, Phyllis, bring her two sons back to our house for dinner. She didn't want to go out and declined the invitation. My father was so mad he had quite a little temper tantrum, and insisted that they come. This was bizarre and unusual behavior for him. Most people would have called him a quiet man with a very dry humor. The temper tantrum impressed Phyllis, so she packed up her two boys and they came over for dinner. Dad drove Phyllis home that evening, but my two cousins stayed the night with us in my brothers' long, dorm-like bedroom.

That night I had an unusual dream. I dreamt I was at a funeral. I could not see any mourners, and I could not see who was in the casket in the corner. A soft light shown down on the room from above, but I could not see the source of the light, either. Dancing under and in the light was a willowy ballerina with a flowing red and white dress. I walked across the room to a table and saw one lone cake with ten fingers sticking out of it like candles. I then suddenly woke up. I knew the dream meant something, but what I was really intrigued with was the fact that I knew in my dream that my grief should have hurt worse than it did.

February Sunday mornings in Wisconsin tend to be cold, dreary, and even dismal. This one was no exception. I remember the moist, dark gray clouds heavy in the sky, and thought it might be a boring, noisy day in our house. The noise, of course, was constant—coming from my four brothers, two cousins, two younger sisters, and the two month-old baby. I was happy and more than a little surprised when Dad suggested he take all of us but the baby to the lake to go sledding for the afternoon. It was cold and ugly, but we were laughing and enjoying ourselves. The only discomfort I remember was thinking I couldn't eat enough snow to quench my thirst. When we were finishing sledding, Dad drove my cousins home and then brought the rest of us to our house, where we mostly scattered to our separate rooms.

My ten and eleven year-old brothers, Perry and Patrick, disappeared outside and were spraying a tread spray on their bike tires. I was forcing myself to do my dreaded bookkeeping homework, when the front door slammed against the wall and

I heard my cousin Todd from next door yell, "Perry's been hit by a car and I think it's bad!"

Perry, at ten years old, was the youngest of my brothers. The next two hours were surreal. I remember jumping up and praying: *God, I don't care if he is alive or dead, but please don't let him suffer.* This was certainly a strange prayer for a girl who had prayed every night that no one in her family would die. Equally strange was the feeling that this prayer had found a home. I usually felt like my prayers went out into the universe and wandered aimlessly around the stars, never reaching their intended target. My parents followed the ambulance to the hospital and I sat watch over my siblings, feeling numb.

About an hour and a half later, a car pulled into the drive, and young man came to the door with a valium prescription. He asked, "Is this the house where the little boy died?"

It's funny, but I suppressed that memory for years before I felt strong enough to let it come to the light of day again.

The next morning my parents went to the funeral home to make arrangements. My five and six year-old sisters asked me if Perry was coming back. I remember looking into their faces and wishing I could give them something to comfort them. These words came from my lips, and I, at least, was comforted: *An egg is a wonderful thing for a growing bird. It nestles inside and is comforted by the safety of the walls around it. As the bird grows, the egg starts to feel tight. One day the shell even begins to crack and the baby bird is scared when the light peeks through. He tries to hold his wings and legs in to keep the shell from cracking some more, but one day it splits wide open and the bird is out in the light and the air. Pretty soon he learns to fly, and he can look down at the broken shell. It feels so good to fly that he would never want to crawl back into that broken, tiny shell again. That is what it is like for Perry. He is in Heaven, and his broken body doesn't look so good to him anymore.*

As it turned out, my siblings were also comforted. I knew that the story did not come from me. It was a gift, but how did I connect with the Giver again? Obviously, loving kindness on His part was the reason for this particular present, but did something this drastic have to happen to hear from Him again?

After the funeral, at which I noted a comforting presence that seemed to blunt my grief, my family returned home to both cry and celebrate. My father's orchestration of one last over-night together, and one last play day as a family, was out of character enough for him that I had to believe a divine hand had pushed him into action. My dream the night before had given my soul a warning that my reasoning mind had not understood, but had somehow let me know that the universe was not surprised by Perry's death.

It seems that my brother Perry had also been dreaming. When my parents went to his school to retrieve the contents of his desk, they found a piece of paper folded up in his pencil case. His teacher was surprised he had not turned it in. The assignment was to write down a recent dream to share. Perry's dream graphically and yet simply described a pig in a farmer's suit driving a red truck. It drove over yards and then hit a big rock. The dream ended with Perry hitting his head and waking up.

In reality, the man who hit Perry was very drunk. Two weeks before he hit Perry, he had been driving a red truck and hit a car parked at a curb, pushing it up and into a yard. I found this out from an extended family member who owned the car. Perry, the French derivative of Peter, means *rock*, as any good Catholic knows. We certainly did. Somehow he knew, deep down, that he was going home.

"Surely the Lord God does nothing
Unless He reveals His secret counsel
To His servants the prophets." Amos 3:7

My brothers did not want to go into the bedroom they had shared with Perry until everything of his had been removed. An aunt and uncle went with me to clean out Perry's things, while my siblings sat together in another room. Next to Perry's bed was a box. In it was his most recent school picture, the sweater he had worn for the picture, and his pocket knife. Why he had packed them up was a mystery at the time, but after reading his dream assignment I understood. I especially liked the wording in the dream: *Then I hit my head and woke up.* I had worried that he might have suffered, even though his broken neck indicated otherwise.

"(3) Blessed be the God and Father of our Lord Jesus Christ, the Father of mercies and God of all comfort, (4) who comforts us in all our affliction so that we will be able to comfort those who are in any affliction with the comfort with which we ourselves are comforted by God."
2 Corinthians 1:3-4

The aforementioned comforting presence continued. I felt it most strongly in our house. Three subdued brothers, two cousins, and one neighbor boy continued to try to do the things boys do, but they didn't laugh much and they all seemed strangely ill at ease with each other. My newest sister, Dana, was five months old, and I believe now that God sent her to us to save us from our grief. We somehow survived the first few months and I have to admit that I don't remember much except the sadness that would ooze from my soul. I have one clear memory of looking in a mirror and thinking, *I want to go home*. Home wasn't the place I was living.

A group of kids from my philosophy class invited me to go to a concert in a nearby city. They were mostly "Jesus freaks" and I didn't really want to go. I always felt that they were judging me to be deficient, often asking if I was "saved." I'm not sure how I ended up going with them; I was probably too weak to put up much of a fight. I arrived to find an auditorium full of people all talking and chatting and looking excited and happy. I felt numb and gray and confused. The "entertainment" walked out onto the stage; evangelists who went by the name of "Sheep." The first thing out of their mouth was, "Everyone is a fool for something or someone. Whose fool are you?"

Was this more judgment? Oddly enough, I really didn't feel that condemned, just thoughtful. I didn't hear what they said for several minutes as I was pondering my place in the world. The next thing I really heard and processed was a beautiful quote from **Matthew 11:28-30**:
> **"(28) "Come to Me, all who are weary and heavy-laden, and I will give you rest.**

(29) Take My yoke upon you and learn from Me, for I am gentle and humble in heart, and you will find rest for your souls. (30) For My yoke is easy and My burden is light."

I don't know how those words broke through the fog of grief surrounding me, but they did. I looked heavenward and said, "Here I am. Take me. Take all of me. I don't want to be in charge of my life and I don't know how to live."

In that moment, a burst of light went off in my head. It was a fraction of a second and I can't explain how I saw it. The same moment I felt unspeakable joy absorb my grief like a great sponge absorbs a few dribbles on the counter. What had become almost unbearably heavy had suddenly become light. It was not my yoke! I had no words or language to describe what had happened that night, but I knew I was not the same girl. My soul craved more. I started reading the Bible for the sheer joy of it. Someone gave me a book, *The Cross and the Switchblade* by David Wilkerson. That was when I discovered that what had happened to me was called being born again. The book was full of stories about miserable, angry, sad people whose lives were transformed.

"...and though you have not seen Him, you love Him, and though you do not see Him now, but

believe in Him, you greatly rejoice with joy inexpressible and full of glory…" 1 Peter 1:8

I shared my great joy with my family. Their initial response was to look confused and try to distance themselves from me. My mother even went so far as to reproach me, saying that she had raised me to be a Christian. Much to her annoyance, I kept talking about the great healing I felt. I tried not to sound preachy, but I am sure that is what they heard. Somehow, in the ensuing years, each one of them had an "aha" moment, when a piece of God's love fell deep into each soul and took root. Eventually, every member of my family was baptized or born again into God's Kingdom.

In hindsight, Perry's death was both heartache and blessing. Who knows if any of us would have even known the joy of our salvation had he not gone home so early? Perhaps we would have each been like my husband, a very good and capable man. So capable, in fact, that he had to endure great disappointment and hardship late in his adulthood before he sought refuge in his Father's heavenly arms.

We will never know how our lives are woven together. I often think of the vision my mom had the night Perry died. She saw two tapestries being woven. One was big and one was little. Both were beautiful. As the tapestries were completed she heard a voice say, "It doesn't matter if it's big or little. When it's finished, it's finished."

Perhaps Perry came here just to lead us to the Father. And then it was finished.

"So teach us to number our days, That we may present to You a heart of wisdom." Psalms 90:12